THE NEW GOITER DIET COOKBOOK

A Practical Nutritional Guide With Simple Recipes For Thyroid-Friendly Living

D1520957

HUDSON DIAZ

2025 by Hudson Diaz .

DISCLAIMER

This publication is intended for informational and educational purposes only. It is not a substitute for professional medical advice, diagnosis, or treatment. Always consult a qualified healthcare provider before making any changes to your diet, especially if you are pregnant, nursing, taking medication, or have any medical condition.

The author and publisher are not responsible for any adverse effects resulting from the use or misuse of the information contained in this book.

LEGAL NOTICE

Contents

CHAPTER 1 5

    Introduction to Goiter and Diet 5

CHAPTER 2 8

    The Basics of the Goiter-Friendly Diet 8

CHAPTER 3 13

    Meal Prep Basics 13

CHAPTER 4 18

    Cooking Procedures and Techniques.....................18

CHAPTER 5 25

    Goiter-Friendly Recipes (Beginner to Advanced)....25

CHAPTER 6 35

    Meal Timing and Portion Control 35

CHAPTER 7 42

    Troubleshooting Common Issues 42

CHAPTER 8 48

    Tips for Staying on Track.......................................48

CONCLUSION 55

CHAPTER 1

Introduction to Goiter and Diet

A goiter is an abnormal enlargement of the thyroid gland, which is located at the base of your neck, just below the Adam's apple. The thyroid is a small butterfly-shaped organ that plays a key role in regulating important bodily functions such as metabolism, energy levels, and body temperature.

When the thyroid becomes enlarged, it can cause swelling in the neck, which can be visible or felt.

Causes of Goiter

Goiter can occur for various reasons, but the most common causes are iodine deficiency and thyroid dysfunction.

1.   Iodine Deficiency: Iodine is an essential mineral that the body needs to make thyroid hormones. When there isn't enough iodine in the diet, the thyroid can't produce enough hormones, leading to an enlargement of the gland. Iodine deficiency is one of the leading causes of goiter around the world, especially in areas where the soil lacks iodine.

2.   Thyroid Dysfunction: Another common cause of goiter is problems with thyroid hormone production. Conditions like hypothyroidism (underactive thyroid) or hyperthyroidism (overactive thyroid) can lead to the enlargement of the thyroid.

In hypothyroidism, the thyroid tries to compensate for the lack of hormone production by growing larger.

Other factors that can contribute to goiter include autoimmune diseases like Graves' disease or Hashimoto's thyroiditis, certain medications, and even pregnancy.

The Role of Diet in Managing Goiter

Diet plays a significant role in managing goiter because it can directly impact thyroid function. By consuming the right foods and avoiding certain foods, it's possible to support thyroid health and, in some cases, reduce the size of a goiter.

1.   Iodine-Rich Foods: Since iodine is essential for thyroid hormone production, adding iodine-rich foods to your diet is crucial for managing goiter. Foods like seafood, iodized salt, and dairy products are excellent sources of iodine.
Including these in your meals can help provide your body with the iodine it needs to support normal thyroid function.

2.   Selenium and Zinc: Selenium and zinc are important minerals that support thyroid health. Brazil nuts, sunflower seeds, and

pumpkin seeds are rich in selenium, while oysters, beef, and chickpeas provide a good source of zinc.

Including these minerals in your diet can help the thyroid function more efficiently.

3. Avoid Goitrogens in Excess: Certain foods, called goitrogens, can interfere with iodine uptake and contribute to thyroid enlargement if consumed in large amounts. These include cruciferous vegetables (like broccoli, cauliflower, and cabbage) and soy-based products. **Cooking these foods can help reduce their goitrogenic effects.**

4. Antioxidants: Antioxidants found in fruits and vegetables can help protect the thyroid from damage caused by inflammation. Foods like berries, spinach, and sweet potatoes are rich in antioxidants and can support overall thyroid health.

CHAPTER 2

The Basics of the Goiter-Friendly Diet

A goiter-friendly diet focuses on foods that support thyroid health and avoid those that may interfere with thyroid function. The goal is to provide the nutrients that your thyroid needs to work properly while minimizing any foods that might make the condition worse.

Beneficial Foods for Goiter Management

1.   Iodine-Rich Foods

Iodine is essential for thyroid hormone production, and a deficiency can contribute to the development of goiter. Including iodine-rich foods in your diet can help support thyroid function.

•   Seafood: Fish such as salmon, tuna, and sardines are excellent sources of iodine.

•   Iodized Salt: Using iodized salt in cooking or on food is an easy way to ensure you are getting enough iodine.

•   Dairy Products: Milk, yogurt, and cheese are good sources of iodine.

•   Seaweed: Seaweed, such as nori, kelp, and wakame, is also a rich source of iodine. You can add it to soups, salads, or sushi.

2.   Selenium

Selenium is a mineral that plays a key role in supporting the thyroid. It helps protect the thyroid from oxidative stress and supports the conversion of thyroid hormones.

•   Brazil Nuts: Just a few Brazil nuts a day provide a healthy dose of selenium.

•   Sunflower Seeds: These are a great, easy-to-snack source of selenium.

•   Eggs: Eggs are another excellent source of selenium, especially the yolk.

•   Mushrooms: These are also rich in selenium and can be added to various dishes.

3.   Zinc

Zinc is essential for proper thyroid function and helps regulate thyroid hormone production.

•   Oysters: These are one of the best sources of zinc.

•   Beef and Lamb: Both are rich in zinc, especially lean cuts.

•   Chickpeas: For a plant-based option, chickpeas (garbanzo beans) are high in zinc.

•   Pumpkin Seeds: These are another great plant-based source of zinc.

4.   Antioxidant-Rich Foods

Antioxidants help protect the thyroid from damage caused by free radicals and inflammation. They also support the overall health of your immune system.

•   Berries: Blueberries, strawberries, and raspberries are packed with antioxidants.

•   Spinach and Kale: Leafy greens are rich in vitamins and antioxidants that support thyroid health.

- Sweet Potatoes: These are rich in beta-carotene, which has antioxidant properties.

- Tomatoes: They provide vitamin C and lycopene, which are beneficial for thyroid protection.

Foods to Avoid

Some foods, while healthy, can interfere with thyroid function when consumed in large amounts. These foods contain substances called goitrogens, which can disrupt iodine absorption and thyroid hormone production. Here are some foods to limit:

1. Soy Products

Soy contains compounds called phytoestrogens that can interfere with thyroid function, especially in people with iodine deficiency. While small amounts of soy may not cause significant issues, it's best to limit foods like tofu, tempeh, and soy milk.

- Example to limit: Tofu, soy milk, soy sauce.

2. Cruciferous Vegetables

Cruciferous vegetables contain substances called glucosinolates, which can interfere with iodine absorption when consumed in large amounts.

These vegetables are healthy but should be eaten in moderation, especially if you have goiter.

•   Examples to limit: Broccoli, cauliflower, cabbage, kale, and Brussels sprouts.

•   Tip: Cooking cruciferous vegetables can help reduce their goitrogenic effect, making them safer to eat.

3.   Excessive Processed Foods

Highly processed foods can often be high in unhealthy fats, sugars, and sodium, which are not beneficial for thyroid health. It's best to focus on whole, nutrient-dense foods.

CHAPTER 3

Meal Prep Basics

Meal prepping is a great way to stay on track with a goiter-friendly diet, especially when you're just starting out. The key to success is planning meals that are easy, nutritious, and fit your dietary needs.

This chapter will walk you through simple and practical steps for planning and preparing goiter-friendly meals, along with tips for saving time and ensuring you have everything you need.

Step 1: Plan Your Meals for the Week

Meal planning is the first step toward a smooth week of healthy eating. Take some time at the start of the week to decide what you will eat for each meal (breakfast, lunch, and dinner).

Here's how to get started:

1.   Choose Goiter-Friendly Meals: Focus on meals that include iodine-rich foods (like seafood and

iodized salt), selenium and zinc-rich foods (like Brazil nuts and eggs), and plenty of antioxidants (from fruits and vegetables). Aim for a balanced diet with proteins, healthy fats, and a variety of vegetables.

Example meals:

- Breakfast: Scrambled eggs with spinach and a side of berries.
- Lunch: Grilled salmon with a mixed greens salad and a sweet potato.
- Dinner: Chicken stir-fry with broccoli, carrots, and brown rice.

2. Make a Variety of Meals: Try to mix things up so you don't get bored with your meals. Prepare a few different protein sources (like chicken, fish, and beans) and a variety of vegetables to ensure you're getting a range of nutrients.

3. Incorporate Leftovers: If you have leftovers from dinner, use them for lunch the next day. This saves time and reduces food waste.

Step 2: Prepare Ingredients in Advance

Preparing ingredients in advance can save a lot of time during the week. By doing some work ahead of time, you'll only need to assemble or cook meals quickly throughout the week.

1. Wash and Chop Vegetables: Wash, peel, and chop vegetables when you have time. Store them in airtight containers in the fridge so they're ready to go when you need them.

o Tip: Pre-cutting vegetables like carrots, bell peppers, and broccoli makes it easy to toss them into stir-fries, salads, or soups.

2. Cook in Batches: Cook large portions of grains (like brown rice or quinoa), proteins (such as chicken or fish), and roasted vegetables all at once. Store them in separate containers in the fridge.

o Example: Roast a whole tray of sweet potatoes and carrots, grill several chicken breasts, and cook a large batch of rice.

3. Prepare Snacks: Pre-portion healthy snacks like nuts, seeds, or fresh fruit. These can be grabbed quickly when you're on the go and help you avoid unhealthy temptations.

4.   Make Sauces and Dressings: Prepare simple dressings, marinades, or sauces in advance, such as a lemon vinaigrette or a yogurt-based dip. Store them in small jars or containers in the fridge.

Step 3: Create a Goiter-Friendly Shopping List

Now that you have a meal plan and know which ingredients to prep, make a shopping list. Keep it simple and stick to the basics.

1.   Focus on Whole Foods: Choose fresh fruits, vegetables, proteins (like poultry, seafood, or legumes), whole grains (brown rice, quinoa), and healthy fats (olive oil, nuts, seeds).

2.   Iodine-Rich Foods: Seafood (like salmon and tuna), iodized salt, dairy products, and seaweed.

3.   Selenium-Rich Foods: Brazil nuts, sunflower seeds, eggs, mushrooms.

4.   Zinc-Rich Foods: Oysters, beef, chickpeas, pumpkin seeds.

5.   Fruits and Vegetables: Fresh berries, spinach, sweet potatoes, tomatoes, kale, and leafy greens. Avoid buying too many cruciferous vegetables or soy products, as they should be limited.

Step 4: Tools and Appliances to Make Meal Prep Easy

Certain kitchen tools and appliances can make meal prepping faster and more efficient. Here are some essentials to have in your kitchen:

1.   Cutting Board and Knives: These are must-have tools for chopping and prepping vegetables and proteins. A sharp knife makes the job easier and safer.

2.   Storage Containers: Invest in good-quality airtight containers to store prepped ingredients and cooked meals. Glass containers are a great option since they are safe for storing food in the fridge and are easy to clean.

3.   Slow Cooker or Instant Pot: These appliances can be a lifesaver when it comes to cooking in batches. Use them to prepare soups, stews, or large amounts of grains and proteins with minimal effort.

4.   Food Processor: If you're chopping large amounts of vegetables, a food processor can save a lot of time. It's also useful for making dressings or chopping nuts and seeds.

5.   Blender: A blender is great for smoothies, making soups, or mixing ingredients for healthy snacks like protein balls.

CHAPTER 4

Cooking Procedures and Techniques

Cooking methods play a key role in preserving the nutrients that support thyroid health. For beginners, it's essential to focus on simple, easy-to-follow techniques that help retain vitamins, minerals, and other important nutrients.

These methods are not only healthy but also easy to use, even for those who are new to cooking.

1. Steaming

Steaming is one of the best cooking methods for retaining the nutrients in food, especially for vegetables. This method uses water vapor to cook food, which helps preserve vitamins and minerals that can be lost during other cooking processes, like boiling.

• Why It's Great for Thyroid Health: Steaming vegetables like spinach, carrots, and broccoli ensures that the thyroid-supporting nutrients like iodine and selenium remain intact.

How to Do It:

- Fill a pot with water, making sure the water doesn't touch the food.
- Place a steaming basket or colander in the pot, and put your vegetables inside.
- Cover the pot with a lid and let the steam cook the food for 5-10 minutes, depending on the size of the vegetables.
- You can also steam fish, chicken, or even eggs in the same way.

• Tip: If you don't have a steaming basket, you can use a metal strainer or sieve, as long as it fits into the pot.

2. Baking

Baking is another great method to preserve nutrients, especially for proteins like chicken, fish, and even vegetables.

It uses dry heat, which helps maintain the flavor and texture of food while keeping the essential nutrients intact.

- Why It's Great for Thyroid Health: Baking doesn't require added fats or oils, making it a healthier choice for maintaining a balanced, thyroid-supporting diet.

How to Do It:

- Preheat your oven to 375°F (190°C).
- Place your protein or vegetables on a baking sheet lined with parchment paper or aluminum foil.
- Season with herbs and spices for extra flavor— try garlic, rosemary, or thyme, which are also good for overall health.
- Bake for 20-30 minutes for chicken or fish, or 40-50 minutes for vegetables, checking for tenderness.

- Tip: When baking fish or chicken, cover the dish with foil for the first half of cooking to keep it moist, then uncover it to brown the top.

3. Grilling

Grilling is a popular cooking method that adds a delicious smoky flavor to food. It's also a quick and healthy way to cook lean proteins and vegetables without using extra fats or oils.

• Why It's Great for Thyroid Health: Grilling helps retain the nutrients of foods like fish and vegetables, while allowing excess fat to drip away.

How to Do It:

- Preheat your grill to medium-high heat.
- For proteins, lightly oil the grill grates to prevent sticking. Place your fish, chicken, or tofu directly on the grill.
- For vegetables like zucchini, bell peppers, and asparagus, toss them with a little olive oil and seasonings before grilling.
- Grill proteins for about 4-6 minutes on each side, depending on thickness. Vegetables should be grilled for 3-5 minutes on each side.

• Tip: If you're new to grilling, try using a grill pan on your stovetop to get the same effect without using an outdoor grill.

4. Sautéing

Sautéing is a quick cooking method that involves cooking food in a small amount of oil or butter over high heat. This technique is great for vegetables, lean proteins, and seafood, as it helps retain their nutrients and natural flavors.

• Why It's Great for Thyroid Health: Sautéing preserves most nutrients, and by using healthy oils like olive oil, you also get the benefit of heart-healthy fats.

How to Do It:

o Heat a pan over medium-high heat and add a small amount of olive oil.

o Once the oil is hot, add your food. Stir it often to avoid burning, and cook until it's tender and lightly browned.

o This method works well for spinach, onions, garlic, and mushrooms, as well as lean cuts of meat like chicken breast or fish fillets.

• Tip: Keep the heat moderate to prevent burning the oil or the food. Stir frequently to ensure even cooking.

5. Boiling and Simmering (In Moderation)

While boiling is not the most nutrient-preserving method, it's still useful for preparing soups or cooking whole grains like quinoa or brown rice. If you're boiling vegetables or grains, avoid overcooking them to prevent nutrient loss.

•　　Why It's Great for Thyroid Health: While some nutrients may leach into the water, boiling is fine for grains and legumes, as they can absorb and retain nutrients during cooking.

•　　**How to Do It:**

- Bring a pot of water to a boil, then reduce to a simmer for gentler cooking.
- For grains or vegetables, cook them in the simmering water until they are tender but not mushy.
- Consider using the cooking water for soups or stews to retain some of the nutrients.

•　　Tip: When boiling vegetables, try to use the smallest amount of water possible to help preserve nutrients.

Tips for Easy and Quick Cooking

1.   Use One-Pot Meals: One-pot meals are an easy way to cook proteins, vegetables, and grains all together. Try dishes like chicken and vegetable stir-fry or a baked salmon with sweet potatoes and spinach.

2.   Batch Cook: Prepare larger portions of your meals at once and store them in the fridge for later. This saves time during the week and makes it easier to stay on track with your goiter-friendly diet.

3.   Use Herbs and Spices: Instead of relying on heavy sauces or oils, use fresh herbs like basil, cilantro, or parsley to add flavor to your dishes. Garlic, turmeric, and ginger are also great for overall health.

CHAPTER 5

Goiter-Friendly Recipes (Beginner to Advanced)

In this chapter, we'll explore a variety of goiter-friendly recipes that range from beginner to advanced. Each recipe is designed to support thyroid health, featuring iodine-rich ingredients, antioxidants, and other essential nutrients.

These easy-to-follow recipes will help you create nutritious and delicious meals, whether you're just starting out or looking to challenge your cooking skills.

Beginner Recipes

1. Simple Iodine-Rich Smoothie

This refreshing smoothie is a quick and easy way to get a healthy dose of iodine, which is essential for managing goiter.

Ingredients:

- 1 cup of unsweetened almond milk (or any dairy-free milk)

- 1/2 banana

- 1/2 cup of spinach

- 1 tablespoon of chia seeds

- 1 tablespoon of honey (optional)

- 1/4 teaspoon of iodized salt

Instructions:

1. Combine the almond milk, banana, spinach, chia seeds, honey, and iodized salt in a blender.

2. Blend until smooth.

3. Pour into a glass and enjoy! You can also add a handful of ice cubes for a colder smoothie.

Why It's Great for Goiter Health: Spinach is packed with antioxidants, while iodized salt provides the necessary iodine to support thyroid function.

2. Baked Salmon with Lemon and Herbs

Salmon is rich in iodine and omega-3 fatty acids, making it a perfect choice for thyroid health.

Ingredients:

•   2 salmon fillets

•   1 tablespoon olive oil

•   1 lemon (sliced)

•   1 teaspoon dried thyme

•   Salt and pepper to taste

•   1 clove garlic (minced)

Instructions:

1.   Preheat your oven to 375°F (190°C).

2.   Place the salmon fillets on a baking sheet lined with parchment paper.

3.	Drizzle the olive oil over the salmon fillets and sprinkle with thyme, salt, pepper, and minced garlic.

4.	Place lemon slices on top of the fillets.

5.	Bake for 15-20 minutes or until the salmon is cooked through and flakes easily with a fork.

6.	Serve with a side of steamed vegetables or a salad.

Why It's Great for Goiter Health: Salmon provides iodine and omega-3s, which help support thyroid function and reduce inflammation.

3. Scrambled Eggs with Iodized Salt

A simple breakfast option that's high in protein and iodine.

Ingredients:

•	2 large eggs

•	1 tablespoon butter or olive oil

•	1/4 teaspoon iodized salt

•	Fresh herbs for garnish (optional)

Instructions:

1.   Crack the eggs into a bowl and whisk them lightly.

2.   Heat butter or olive oil in a non-stick pan over medium heat.

3.   Pour the eggs into the pan and cook, stirring occasionally, until they are softly scrambled.

4.   Sprinkle with iodized salt and garnish with fresh herbs if desired.

5.   Serve warm with a side of whole-grain toast.

Why It's Great for Goiter Health: Eggs are a great source of protein and iodine. Using iodized salt boosts your iodine intake in a simple way.

Intermediate Recipes

1. Miso Soup with Seaweed

This nourishing soup is full of iodine from the seaweed and offers an umami-rich flavor.

Ingredients:

•   4 cups water

- 2 tablespoons miso paste (choose a low-sodium variety)

- 1/2 cup dried seaweed (wakame)

- 1/2 cup tofu (cubed)

- 1 green onion (chopped)

Instructions:

1. Bring the water to a boil in a medium saucepan.

2. Stir in the miso paste until it dissolves completely.

3. Add the dried seaweed and tofu to the pot and simmer for 5-7 minutes.

4. Stir in the chopped green onions before serving.

5. Ladle the soup into bowls and enjoy warm.

Why It's Great for Goiter Health: Seaweed is an excellent natural source of iodine, and miso adds a savory flavor while providing probiotics for gut health.

2. Thyroid-Boosting Salad

A nutrient-packed salad filled with goiter-friendly ingredients like spinach, sunflower seeds, and avocado.

Ingredients:

- 2 cups fresh spinach

- 1/2 avocado (sliced)

- 1 tablespoon sunflower seeds

- 1/4 cup shredded carrots

- 1 tablespoon olive oil

- 1 teaspoon apple cider vinegar

- Salt and pepper to taste

Instructions:

1. In a large bowl, combine the spinach, avocado slices, sunflower seeds, and shredded carrots.

2. Drizzle with olive oil and apple cider vinegar, and toss to combine.

3. Season with salt and pepper to taste.

4.   Serve immediately as a side dish or a light lunch.

Why It's Great for Goiter Health: Spinach is rich in antioxidants, and sunflower seeds provide selenium, a vital nutrient for thyroid health.

Advanced Recipes

1. Quinoa Salad with Seafood

This advanced dish combines quinoa, seafood, and vegetables into a flavorful and nutrient-rich meal.

Ingredients:

- 1 cup quinoa (rinsed)

- 2 cups water or vegetable broth

- 1/2 pound shrimp (peeled and deveined)

- 1/2 pound cooked lobster (optional)

- 1 cup cherry tomatoes (halved)

- 1/4 cup fresh parsley (chopped)

- 1 tablespoon olive oil

- 1 tablespoon lemon juice

- Salt and pepper to taste

Instructions:

1. Cook the quinoa: Bring 2 cups of water or broth to a boil in a medium saucepan. Add the quinoa, reduce the heat, and cover. Simmer for 15 minutes, or until the water is absorbed and the quinoa is tender.

2. In a separate pan, sauté the shrimp in olive oil over medium heat for 3-4 minutes per side, until they turn pink.

3. In a large bowl, combine the cooked quinoa, shrimp, lobster, cherry tomatoes, and parsley.

4. Drizzle with olive oil and lemon juice, then season with salt and pepper to taste.

5. Toss everything together and serve warm or chilled.

Why It's Great for Goiter Health: Quinoa is a complete protein, and seafood is rich in iodine and selenium, both essential for thyroid health.

2. Stuffed Sweet Potatoes with Spinach

This hearty and nutrient-dense recipe offers a satisfying meal with thyroid-supporting ingredients.

Ingredients:

- 4 medium sweet potatoes

- 2 cups fresh spinach

- 1 tablespoon olive oil

- 1 clove garlic (minced)

- 1/4 cup feta cheese (optional)

- Salt and pepper to taste

Instructions:

1.   Preheat your oven to 400°F (200°C).

2.   Pierce the sweet potatoes with a fork and bake them for 45-50 minutes, until tender.

3.   While the potatoes bake, heat olive oil in a pan and sauté the garlic for 1-2 minutes. Add the spinach and cook until wilted, about 3-4 minutes.

4.   Once the sweet potatoes are done, cut a slit down the center of each and gently fluff the insides with a fork.

5.   Stuff the potatoes with the sautéed spinach and garlic mixture. Top with feta cheese, salt, and pepper to taste.

6.   Serve warm and enjoy!

CHAPTER 6

Meal Timing and Portion Control

In managing goiter, the timing and portion control of your meals are just as important as the types of food you eat. Understanding how meal timing impacts thyroid function and digestion can make a significant difference in your overall health.

In this chapter, we will explore how to optimize meal timing and portion sizes to support thyroid health while making it easy for beginners to follow.

The Importance of Meal Timing for Thyroid Health

Meal timing is essential for regulating thyroid function and maintaining steady energy levels. The thyroid gland controls metabolism, so eating at regular intervals helps support its role in regulating hormones and energy production.]

Eating smaller, balanced meals throughout the day can help avoid spikes or dips in energy that might lead to overeating or undereating, both of which can stress the thyroid.

Why Meal Timing Matters for Goiter:

•   Consistent Energy Levels: Eating at regular intervals prevents blood sugar crashes, which can affect thyroid function.

•   Improved Digestion: Spacing meals out allows your body to better digest and absorb the nutrients it needs without feeling overwhelmed.

•   Hormonal Balance: A regular eating schedule can help maintain the balance of thyroid hormones, preventing sudden fluctuations.

Best Times to Eat for Thyroid Health

To support your thyroid, aim for three main meals a day, along with one or two small snacks in between. This routine helps maintain a steady flow of nutrients to your body while giving your thyroid the consistent energy it needs to function properly.

• Breakfast (Within 1 hour of waking up): Starting your day with a nutritious breakfast is essential for jump-starting metabolism and providing your body with the energy it needs to function throughout the day.

Include protein-rich foods like eggs or yogurt, and incorporate iodine-rich foods like iodized salt or seaweed.

• Lunch (Midday, 4-5 hours after breakfast): A balanced lunch with lean protein, whole grains, and vegetables can support steady thyroid hormone production. Keep portion sizes moderate to avoid feeling sluggish afterward.

• Dinner (5-6 hours after lunch): For dinner, keep the meal light yet satisfying to prevent overeating before bedtime. Avoid eating too late to ensure proper digestion.

Focus on vegetables, lean proteins, and healthy fats like olive oil or avocado.

• Snacks (Optional, 2-3 hours after meals): If you feel hungry between meals, opt for small, balanced snacks such as nuts, fruits, or a small portion of yogurt. Avoid sugary snacks or large portions that can lead to overeating.

Portion Control: How Much Should You Eat?

Portion control is key to managing goiter. Eating the right amount of food—enough to nourish the body without overloading the digestive system—is important for thyroid health.

 Overeating can lead to weight gain and stress the thyroid, while undereating may leave the body lacking vital nutrients that support thyroid function.

Here are some tips for portion control:

•   Use the Plate Method: Fill half of your plate with vegetables, one-quarter with lean protein (such as fish, chicken, or tofu), and the remaining quarter with whole grains or starchy vegetables (like sweet potatoes or quinoa).

•   Smaller, More Frequent Meals: Instead of eating large portions at once, try eating smaller meals throughout the day. This helps keep your energy levels steady and supports digestion.

•   Listen to Your Body: Pay attention to hunger and fullness cues. Eating slowly and savoring your food helps you recognize when you're full, preventing overeating.

•   Measure Portions for Beginners: When you're just starting out, measuring portions can help you understand how much food is appropriate.

For example, a serving of protein should be roughly the size of your palm, and a serving of grains or starchy vegetables should be about the size of your fist.

Benefits of Smaller, Balanced Meals Throughout the Day

For those with goiter, eating smaller, balanced meals throughout the day offers several advantages:

1.   Stable Thyroid Function: Smaller meals prevent large fluctuations in blood sugar, which can affect thyroid hormones. This steady intake helps your thyroid function more efficiently.

2.   Better Digestion: Eating smaller meals reduces the risk of digestive discomfort, as the body doesn't have to process large quantities of food at once.

This also allows better absorption of nutrients that support thyroid health.

3.   Prevention of Overeating or Undereating: By sticking to regular meal times and portion sizes, you can avoid the negative impacts of overeating (which can lead to weight gain and stress on the thyroid) or undereating (which can deprive the thyroid of essential nutrients).

4.   Improved Energy Levels: With consistent meal timing, your energy levels will remain more stable throughout the day, reducing fatigue and helping you stay active and alert.

Practical Tips for Beginners

1.   Plan Your Meals Ahead of Time: Preparing meals in advance ensures you always have balanced, portion-controlled options on hand, making it easier to stick to your meal schedule.

2.   Use a Timer or Reminder: If you're new to meal timing, setting reminders on your phone or a kitchen timer can help you stay on track with eating at regular intervals.

3.   Keep Healthy Snacks Available: Having goiter-friendly snacks readily available, like nuts, fruit, or yogurt, will make it easier to stick to portion control and avoid unhealthy choices.

4.   Start Small: If you're not used to smaller meals, start by gradually reducing portion sizes and adding more meals throughout the day. This will help your body adjust without feeling overwhelmed.

CHAPTER 7

Troubleshooting Common Issues

Following a goiter-friendly diet can sometimes come with challenges, especially in the beginning. You may face difficulties staying consistent, dealing with cravings for foods that aren't recommended, or experiencing some side effects as your body adjusts to new eating habits.

In this chapter, we'll address common issues that people encounter and provide practical solutions to help you stay on track while supporting thyroid health.

1. Staying Consistent with Your Diet

Staying consistent with your goiter-friendly diet is key to seeing the positive effects on your thyroid health. However, maintaining consistency can be tricky, especially when life gets busy or when you're tempted to fall back into old eating habits.

Tips for Consistency:

• Plan Your Meals: The more you plan ahead, the easier it is to stay consistent. Take some time each week to plan your meals, create a shopping list, and prep as much as you can in advance.

This will save time during the week and help you avoid making last-minute, unhealthy food choices.

• Set Realistic Goals: Don't expect perfection. It's okay to make mistakes or slip up occasionally. Focus on progress, not perfection. Start with small, achievable changes and build on them over time.

• Track Your Progress: Keep a food journal or use a meal-tracking app to monitor what you eat and how you feel. This will help you stay motivated and spot patterns that may need adjusting.

• Get Support: Share your goals with a friend or family member who can help keep you accountable. You could even join an online community or support group where others are following a similar diet.

2. Dealing with Cravings for Goiter-Unfriendly Foods

Cravings for foods that aren't part of a goiter-friendly diet, such as soy products, processed snacks, or cruciferous vegetables, are common.

It's normal to miss certain foods, but there are ways to manage these cravings without giving up on your diet.

Strategies for Handling Cravings:

•	Find Substitutes: Try to find goiter-friendly alternatives that satisfy your cravings. For example, if you miss a hearty serving of soy-based food, consider trying a small portion of iodine-rich seafood or beans instead.

•	Eat Balanced Meals: Ensure your meals are satisfying and nutrient-dense. Sometimes, cravings are simply the result of not feeling full or not getting enough nutrients. Including healthy fats, proteins, and fiber in every meal will help you feel full and satisfied.

•	Mindful Eating: Practice mindful eating by taking the time to enjoy your meals and focus on how your body feels. Slow down, savor the flavors, and avoid overeating or reaching for unhealthy foods out of habit.

•   Allow Occasional Treats: If you're craving something specific, it's okay to enjoy it occasionally in moderation, but try to limit it. Having a small portion of a goiter-unfriendly food now and then can help satisfy the craving without derailing your progress.

3. Managing Potential Side Effects of Dietary Changes

When you change your diet, it's normal for your body to go through an adjustment period.

You may experience some side effects as your body adapts to new foods, especially if you're introducing more iodine-rich or nutrient-dense foods into your meals.

Common Side Effects and How to Manage Them:

•   Digestive Discomfort: As you start eating more fiber-rich foods like vegetables, whole grains, and legumes, your digestive system might need time to adjust. If you experience bloating or discomfort, try to increase fiber gradually and drink plenty of water to help your digestive system adjust.

• Energy Fluctuations: It's common to feel more tired than usual when changing your eating habits, especially if you've reduced your intake of processed foods or sugar.

Give your body time to adapt, and focus on balanced meals that provide steady energy throughout the day.

• Possible Detox Symptoms: As your body adjusts to a healthier diet, you may experience symptoms like headaches or mild fatigue. This can be part of the detox process as your body rids itself of excess toxins. Stay hydrated, get enough rest, and be patient with yourself.

4. Staying Motivated Throughout the Process

It can be difficult to stay motivated when you're not immediately seeing results. However, it's important to remember that making changes to your diet is a long-term commitment, and the benefits may take time to show.

Staying motivated can be challenging, but with the right mindset and strategies, it's possible to keep moving forward.

Tips for Staying Motivated:

• Celebrate Small Wins: Focus on small victories along the way. Whether it's feeling more energized, reducing inflammation, or simply sticking to your meal plan for the week, celebrate your progress.

• Remind Yourself of Your Why: Keep a reminder of why you started this journey. Whether it's to improve your thyroid health, feel better overall, or prevent the goiter from worsening, keeping your "why" in mind can help you stay focused.

• Track Your Improvements: While it might take some time to see physical changes, track other improvements like better digestion, improved energy, or clearer skin. These positive changes can keep you motivated and excited to continue.

• Stay Flexible: Life is full of unexpected events, and it's okay if things don't always go as planned. If you miss a meal or can't follow your diet perfectly for a day or two, don't be hard on yourself.

Just get back on track and keep moving forward.

CHAPTER 8

Tips for Staying on Track

Adopting a goiter-friendly diet is an important step toward supporting your thyroid health. However, like any lifestyle change, sticking with it can be challenging. This chapter provides practical tips for beginners to stay motivated and consistent with their new eating habits.

We'll focus on creating a daily routine, overcoming obstacles, and celebrating small successes to keep you on track as you work toward better health.

1. Create a Daily Routine

Having a structured daily routine can make it much easier to stick to your goiter-friendly diet. When you plan your day around your meals and dietary needs, it reduces the chances of feeling overwhelmed or falling off track. Here's how to build a routine that works for you:

•   Meal Prep in Advance: One of the easiest ways to stay consistent is to plan your meals ahead of time. Set aside a day each week (like Sunday) to prepare meals for the upcoming days.

 This can include chopping vegetables, cooking grains like quinoa or rice, or portioning out proteins like fish or chicken.

Having meals ready to go reduces the temptation to grab unhealthy options when you're hungry and pressed for time.

•   Set Regular Meal Times: Try to eat at consistent times each day. This will help regulate your metabolism and prevent overeating or skipping meals. Having regular meal times also supports thyroid function by keeping your energy levels steady.

•   Incorporate Mindfulness Practices: Mindful eating involves paying attention to how you feel before, during, and after meals. Take the time to enjoy your food, savor the flavors, and listen to your body's hunger and fullness cues.

Mindfulness practices like meditation, deep breathing, or even a short walk before meals can help reduce stress and keep you centered throughout the day.

2. Overcoming Challenges

No diet is without challenges, and it's common to feel frustrated or tempted to give up at times. However, with the right mindset, you can overcome these obstacles and stay on track.

Common Challenges and Solutions:

• Temptation from Non-Goiter-Friendly Foods: If you're craving foods that aren't part of your diet, try finding healthier alternatives that satisfy the craving. For example, if you miss a sweet snack, try fresh fruit or a small portion of dark chocolate.

Keep goiter-friendly snacks on hand to avoid temptation.

• Time Constraints: Life can get busy, and sometimes cooking feels like a chore. On these days, consider batch-cooking your meals or using a slow cooker to prepare meals that require little effort.

You can also prep quick meals like salads, smoothies, or scrambled eggs with iodine-rich foods that only take a few minutes.

•   Feeling Overwhelmed: If you're just starting out, it can be easy to feel overwhelmed by all the new information and changes. Start small by focusing on one or two meals a day, and gradually build up to full-day meal plans.

Don't rush the process—progress is more important than perfection.

3. Stay Organized

Being organized can help you stay focused and reduce stress when following your goiter-friendly diet. A little preparation goes a long way toward ensuring you stick to your new eating habits.

•   Use a Meal Planner: Invest in a meal planner or use an app to track your meals. This will help you see what you've eaten and plan your upcoming meals. It also helps to avoid the stress of deciding what to eat last minute.

•   Grocery List and Shopping: Keep a grocery list that includes all the goiter-friendly foods you'll need for the week. Having a list prevents impulse buys and ensures you stay stocked up on healthy foods that support thyroid health.

• Keep Your Kitchen Stocked: Make sure your pantry and fridge are stocked with goiter-friendly ingredients. Having easy access to iodine-rich foods like seafood, dairy, and iodized salt, as well as selenium and zinc-rich foods like nuts and seeds, will make it easier to stick to your diet.

4. Celebrate Small Wins

Staying motivated is easier when you acknowledge and celebrate your progress. While the goal is to improve thyroid health, it's also important to celebrate the small victories along the way.

• Track Your Progress: Keep a journal or a log of how you're feeling throughout the process. Record any improvements you notice, whether it's feeling more energized, experiencing less bloating, or noticing a reduction in the size of your goiter.

• Set Mini Goals: Break down your overall goal into smaller, achievable targets. For example, aim to stick to your meal prep routine for one week, or try incorporating a new goiter-friendly food into your diet. Celebrate these mini achievements to stay motivated.

•	Reward Yourself (in Healthy Ways): After accomplishing a goal, treat yourself to something that supports your wellness journey. This could be a relaxing activity like a bath, a walk in nature, or a yoga class. It's important to reward yourself in a way that reinforces your commitment to health.

5. Seek Additional Resources and Support

Sometimes, you may need extra encouragement to stay on track. There are many resources available that can offer guidance, support, and motivation.

•	Books and Cookbooks: There are many cookbooks and online resources specifically designed for thyroid health. These can provide new recipe ideas, helpful tips, and additional support to keep you excited about your diet.

•	Online Communities: Consider joining an online group or forum where others are also following a goiter-friendly diet. Sharing experiences, recipes, and success stories can help you stay motivated and provide answers to any questions you have along the way.

• Consult a Dietitian or Nutritionist: If you need personalized guidance, consider consulting a registered dietitian who specializes in thyroid health. They can help tailor your diet to your specific needs and ensure you're getting the nutrients your thyroid requires.

CONCLUSION

Congratulations on taking the first step toward supporting your thyroid health through a goiter-friendly diet! By reading this book and implementing the tips, recipes, and strategies shared, you are setting yourself up for long-term success.

Remember, the journey toward better health is a process, and it's important to stay patient and persistent as you adapt to your new eating habits.

Small, consistent changes—whether it's introducing more iodine-rich foods, experimenting with new recipes, or simply being mindful of portion sizes—can have a significant, positive impact on your thyroid health over time.

It's the small daily choices that add up to lasting improvements.

As you continue to explore and refine your goiter-friendly diet, keep in mind that it's okay to take things one step at a time. There will be challenges along the way, but each step forward is a victory. Stay motivated and give yourself credit for the progress you make, no matter how small it may seem.

If you ever find yourself uncertain or facing difficulties, don't hesitate to seek professional guidance. A nutritionist, dietitian, or healthcare provider specializing in thyroid health can offer personalized support to help you optimize your diet further.

Their expertise can provide valuable insights tailored to your specific needs.

Above all, stay focused on your well-being and the positive changes you're making. Your commitment to a goiter-friendly lifestyle is a powerful step toward better health, and every effort you put in is worth it. With patience, persistence, and the right tools, you'll see the benefits of your hard work and create a healthier, more vibrant life.

A

Made in United States
North Haven, CT
06 May 2025

68630364R00036